first book of
horses
and ponies

Isabel Thomas

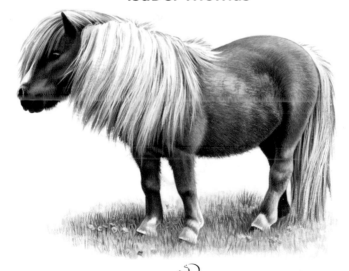

A & C BLACK
AN IMPRINT OF BLOOMSBURY
LONDON NEW DELHI NEW YORK SYDNEY

Published 2014 by
A&C Black
An imprint of Bloomsbury Publishing Plc
50 Bedford Square, London, WC1B 3DP

www.bloomsbury.com

ISBN 978-1-4729-0399-0

This book is produced using paper that is made from wood
grown in managed, sustainable forests. It is natural, renewable
and recyclable. The logging and manufacturing processes
conform to the environmental regulations of the country of origin.

Printed in China by Leo Paper Products, Heshan, Guangdong

10 9 8 7 6 5 4 3 2 1

Horse and pony safety

Always have an adult with you when you look at
horses and ponies. Some of these animals can be
frightened by loud noises. Keep quiet and move
slowly when you are near horses and ponies.

Contents

Horses and ponies

Horses and ponies are amazing animals. They have helped people to do important jobs for thousands of years. People also ride horses and ponies for fun and for sport.

This book will help you to name the different breeds you see. It tells you whether they are horses or ponies. The main difference between horses and ponies is their height. Ponies measure less than 14.2 hands (142 cm). Some horses are as small as ponies, but are called horses because of their body shape, or the way they behave.

At the back of this book is a Spotter's Guide to help you remember the horses and ponies you spot. Tick the breeds off as you see them. You can also find out the meaning of some useful horse and pony words.

Turn the page to find out all about horses and ponies!

Akhal-Teke (horse)

This is one of the oldest breeds of horse in the world. Akhal-Tekes are famous for being fast and strong. They are very good at racing.

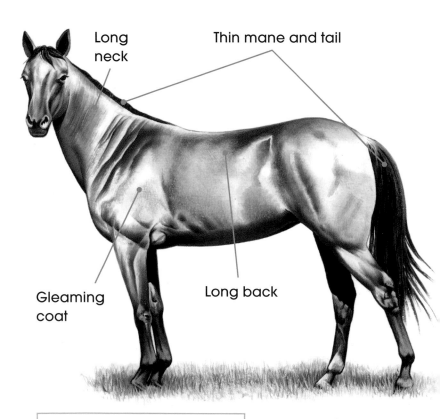

Long neck

Thin mane and tail

Gleaming coat

Long back

The Akhal-Teke's coat gleams like gold in sunlight.

American Saddlebred (horse)

addlebreds are the most popular riding
orses in the USA. They are famous all
round the world for
heir great performances in
orse shows.

Saddlebreds
have starred
in several
Hollywood
films.

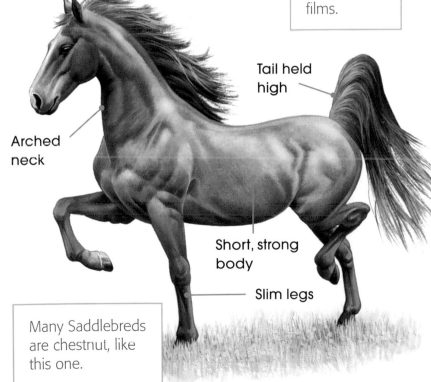

Tail held
high

Arched
neck

Short, strong
body

Slim legs

Many Saddlebreds
are chestnut, like
this one.

Andalucian (horse)

This is a famous Spanish horse. Most Andalucians are grey, but they can also be bay, black, and roan. They are fast, brave, and easy to train.

Long mane and forelock

Crest on neck

Strong shoulders

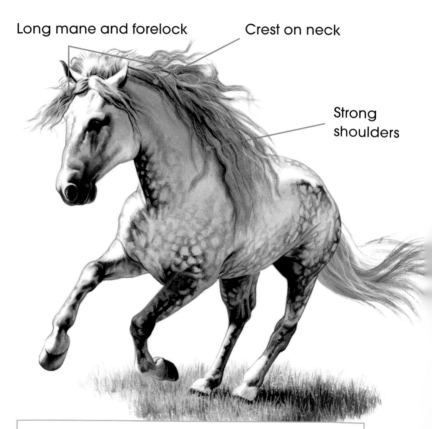

European kings once rode Andalucians to go into battle. They were known as the Horse of Kings.

Appaloosa (horse)

Appaloosas are popular riding horses. Their coats can have six different patterns. To spot an Appaloosa, look for mottled pink and black skin around the nose and eyes.

The Appaloosa patterns are called snowflake, leopard, frost, marble, spotted blanket, and white blanket.

Mottled skin around nose and eyes

Grey coat

Roan spots

Black and white stripes on hooves

This leopard Appaloosa is taking part in a rodeo.

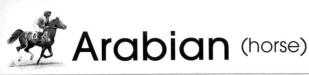

Arabian (horse)

Arabian horses are the world's most famous horses. They are beautiful and very fast. Spot them speeding around racetracks.

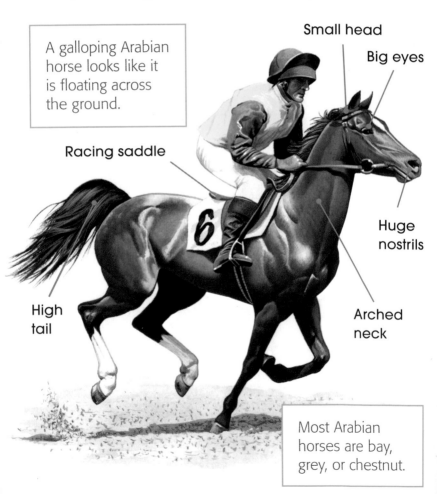

A galloping Arabian horse looks like it is floating across the ground.

Small head

Big eyes

Racing saddle

Huge nostrils

High tail

Arched neck

Most Arabian horses are bay, grey, or chestnut.

Ardennes (horse)

These massive horses once worked on farms. They did all the jobs that tractors do today. Ardennes horses are still used to pull very heavy loads.

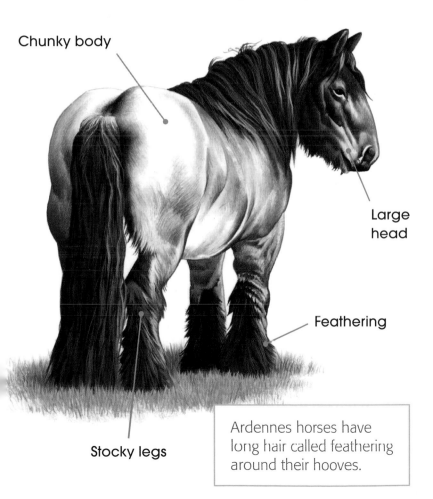

Chunky body

Large head

Feathering

Stocky legs

Ardennes horses have long hair called feathering around their hooves.

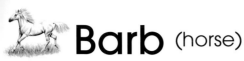

Barb (horse)

These tough horses come from deserts in North Africa. They can run very fast in short races. Barbs are also famous for being quite bad-tempered.

Arabian and Camargue horses both look very similar to Barbs.

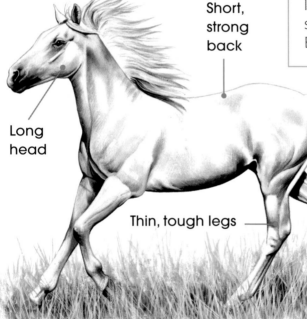

Short, strong back

Long head

Thin, tough legs

Small feet

Many other breeds of horses are related to Barbs.

Camargue (small horse)

Grey Camargue horses live in a swampy national park in France. They have roamed free here for thousands of years.

Camargue foals are black or brown. They turn grey when they are about four years old.

Sometimes cowboys ride Camargue horses, to help round up black bulls.

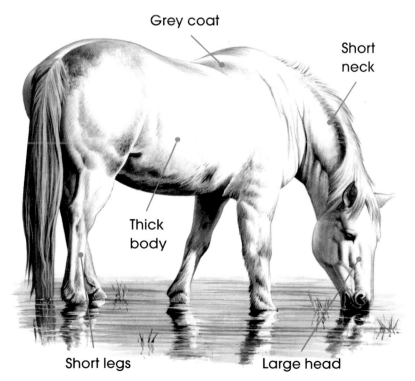

Grey coat

Short neck

Thick body

Short legs

Large head

Caspian (small horse)

These miniature horses come from Iran. They are small but speedy. Thousands of years ago, a Persian king used Caspians to pull his chariot on lion hunts.

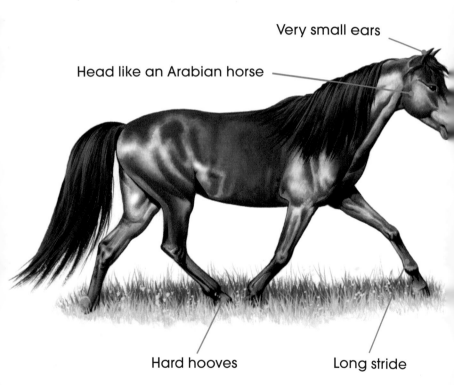

Very small ears

Head like an Arabian horse

Hard hooves

Long stride

Today, Caspians are popular horses for children to ride.

Cleveland Bay (horse)

Clevelands are the horses that pull the carriages of the British Royal Family. Look out for them at equestrian sports events like dressage and showjumping.

All Cleveland Bays are the same colour.

Large head

Small white star

Thick, muscled neck

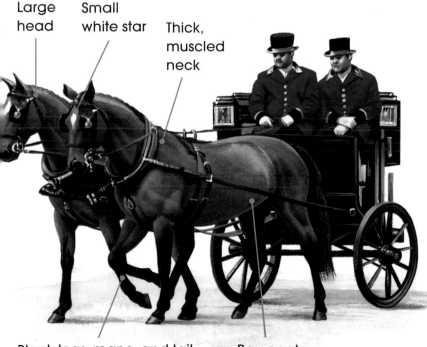

Black legs, mane, and tail

Bay coat

Clydesdale (horse)

These giant horses were bred to pull heavy loads around farms in Scotland. They were so good at their job, they were sent around the world. Now you can spot them everywhere from New Zealand to Hawaii.

Clydesdales may be huge, but they move with quick, springy strides.

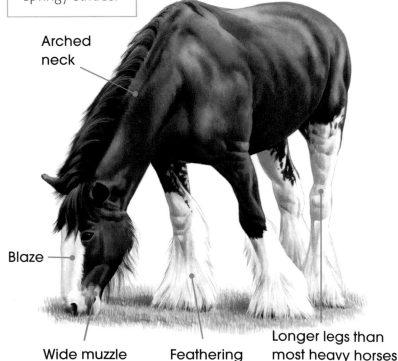

Arched neck

Blaze

Wide muzzle

Feathering

Longer legs than most heavy horses

Connemara (pony)

Look out for Connemara ponies working at riding schools. Many children learn to ride on these calm and friendly ponies.

The first Connemara ponies lived on moorlands in Ireland.

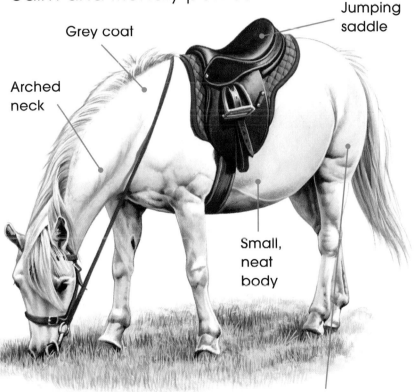

Grey coat

Arched neck

Jumping saddle

Small, neat body

Powerful hindquarters

Connemara ponies are great at showjumping.

Dartmoor (pony)

Dartmoor ponies come from Devon, England. You can still spot them roaming across the moorland. Dartmoor ponies are also popular show ponies.

The ponies that live on Dartmoor are not wild. They all have owners.

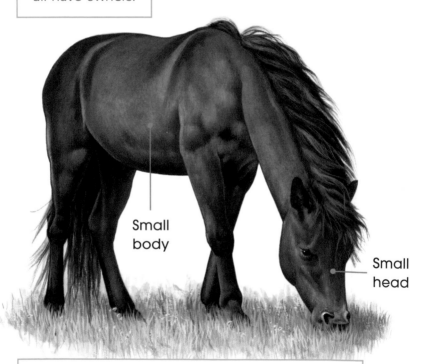

Small body

Small head

Some horses and ponies sleep for just two hours a day. They spend the rest of the time eating.

Exmoor (pony)

Exmoor ponies are very rare. Just a few hundred still live on Exmoor in Devon, England. They have strong teeth to chomp through tough grass and spiky gorse.

Exmoor ponies have 'toad eyes'. Their eyelids are shaped like hoods, to keep out wind and rain.

Toad eye

Mealy muzzle

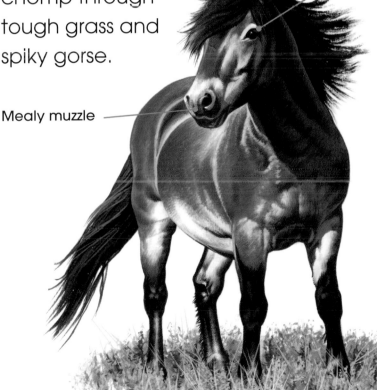

Falabella (small horse)

Falabellas are the world's smallest horses. They are less than a metre tall. They may be tiny but they are tough. They can pull small carriages and carry children.

The first Falabella horses came from Argentina in South America. Now you can spot them around the world.

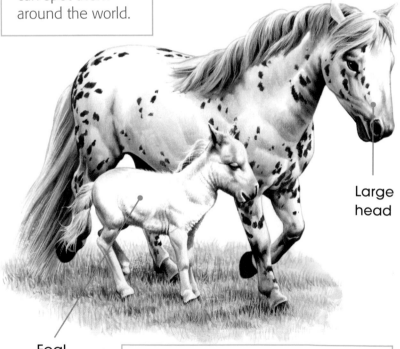

Large head

Foal

Falabellas are called miniature horses.

Fell (pony)

Fell ponies are tough and strong. Before railways were invented, they were used to pull heavy loads from

> Most Fell ponies are black.
> They can look like miniature Friesian horses.

place to place. Today, you can spot Fell ponies taking part in a sport called driving.

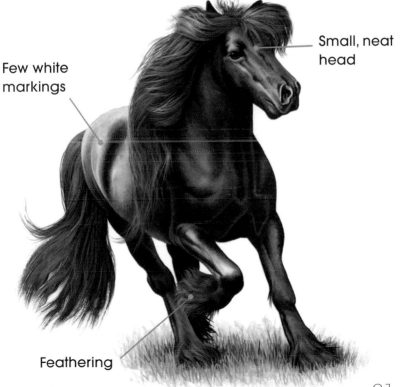

Small, neat head

Few white markings

Feathering

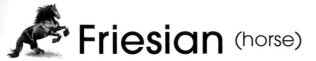

Friesian (horse)

In the past, knights often rode Friesians. These beautiful black horses could trot quickly, even carrying heavy suits of armour. Today, you might spot Friesians working together to pull carriages in competitions.

Some Friesians have a small white star on their forehead.

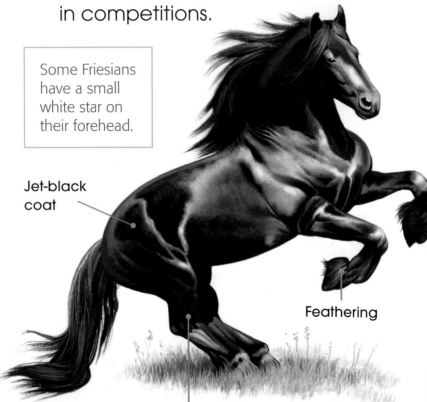

Jet-black coat

Feathering

Short, strong legs

Gotland (pony)

These ponies come from the island of Gotland in Sweden. In the past, Gotland ponies were rounded up to work on farms. Now thousands of them live in the wild again.

In Sweden, the Gotland is called 'little horse of the woods' or 'little goat'.

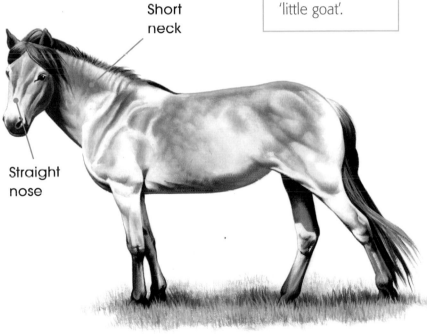

Short neck

Straight nose

Gotlands are gentle and friendly ponies.

Hackney Horse (horse)

Hackney Horses love to show off! Look out for their amazing high-stepping trot at horse shows. They have very bendy joints. You might spot Hackney Ponies too.

Before cars and trucks were invented, horses were the only way to move people and things from place to place.

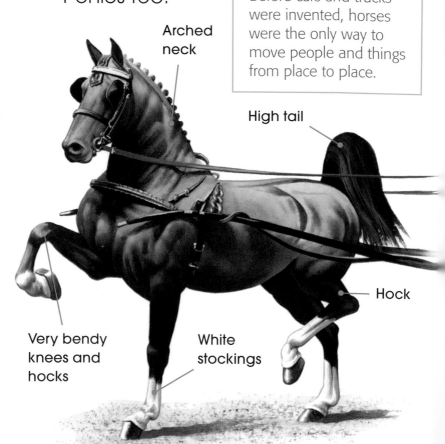

Arched neck

High tail

Hock

Very bendy knees and hocks

White stockings

Haflinger (pony)

Nearly all Haflingers have chestnut coats,

> The world's first Haflinger was called Follie.

and a flaxen mane and tail. They are friendly ponies. Look out for them at riding schools and shows.

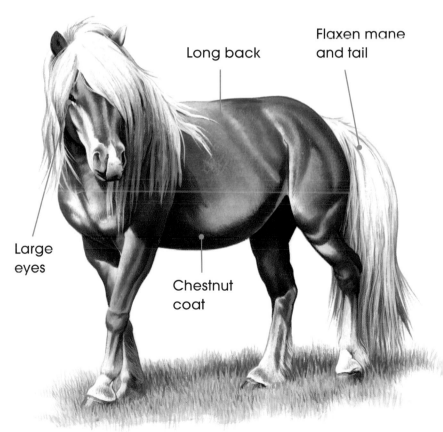

Long back

Flaxen mane and tail

Large eyes

Chestnut coat

Hanoverian (horse)

These famous German horses are brilliant at dressage and showjumping. They look very graceful as they fly over fences. Look out for the H-shaped marks on their hips.

Hanoverians take a special test before they have foals. Only the foals of parents who pass are called Hanoverians.

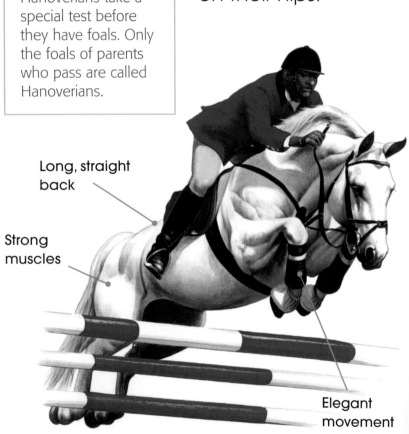

Long, straight back

Strong muscles

Elegant movement

Highland (pony)

These ponies come from the highlands of Scotland. The weather can get very bad there, so Highland Ponies grow a thick winter coat. Highland ponies can be many different colours.

Highland Ponies are used for pony trekking. They are also good at jumping and dressage.

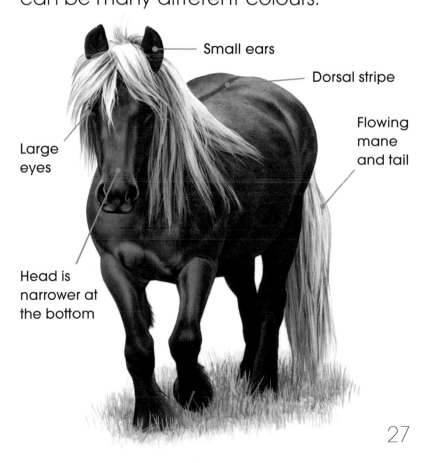

Small ears

Dorsal stripe

Flowing mane and tail

Large eyes

Head is narrower at the bottom

Icelandic Horse (pony)

The Icelandic Horse is really a pony. It has a special walk called the tölt (pronounced 'tolt'). This is a walk that is as fast as a run. The tölt is very comfortable for the rider.

Icelandic Horses are the only kind of horse or pony that live in Iceland.

Double-sided mane

Large head

Lipizzaner (horse)

Lipizzaners perform at the famous Spanish Riding School of Vienna. This is like a ballet school for horses. The horses learn how to do perfect movements. They get sugar lumps as a reward.

Most Lipizzaners are white-grey. A few are bay.

Large head

Snowy-white coat

Strong legs

Lipizzaner foals are born dark brown or black. They change colour as they grow.

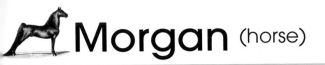 # Morgan (horse)

Morgans are very popular riding horses in the USA. They are said to be clever, calm, charming, and good at everything.

The first Morgan was a famous horse called Figure. His name was changed to Justin Morgan, after his owner.

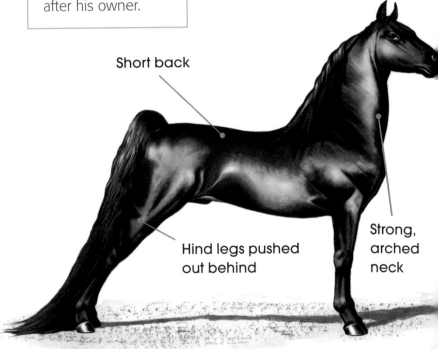

Short back

Hind legs pushed out behind

Strong, arched neck

Percheron (horse)

These heavy horses come from France, but you can spot them all around the world. Some work on farms, helping with jobs such as ploughing. Others are used for riding.

Percherons are very calm horses and are not upset by loud noises.

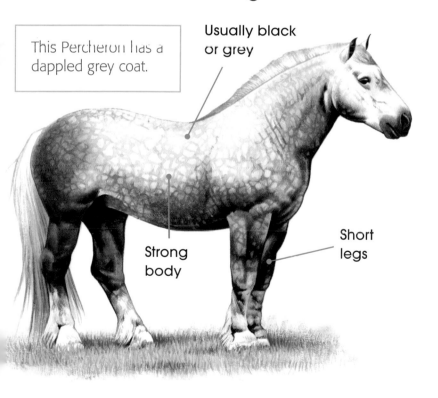

This Percheron has a dappled grey coat.

Usually black or grey

Strong body

Short legs

Pony of the Americas (pony)

These ponies have coats with spotted patterns, like Appaloosa horses. They are gentle and easy to train. This makes them great for children to ride.

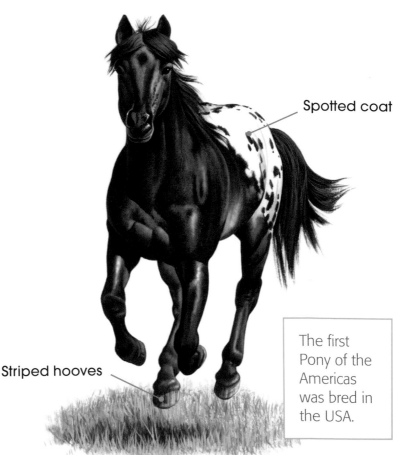

Spotted coat

Striped hooves

The first Pony of the Americas was bred in the USA.

Przewalski's Horse (small horse)

Thousands of years ago, the only horses were wild horses like Przewalski's Horse. More than 300 of these horses still roam around huge grasslands in Asia. You can also spot them in zoos and wildlife parks.

Pictures of horses like this were painted on cave walls 20,000 years ago.

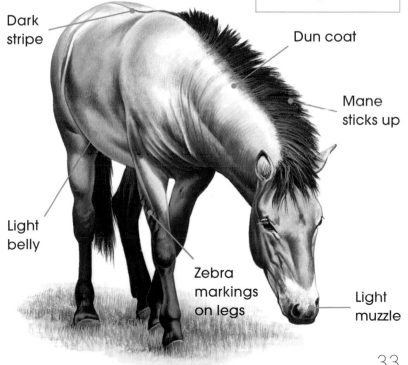

Dark stripe

Dun coat

Mane sticks up

Light belly

Zebra markings on legs

Light muzzle

Quarter Horse (horse)

Millions of Quarter Horses are kept all around the world. They are popular because they are good at everything!

Quarter Horses are named after a quarter-mile race. These speedy horses can't be beaten.

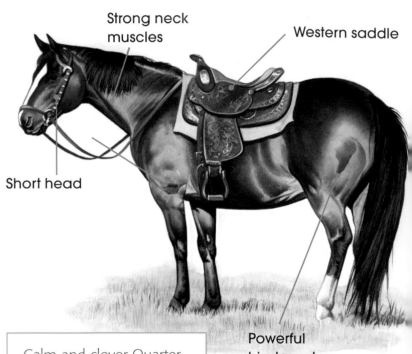

Strong neck muscles

Western saddle

Short head

Powerful hindquarters

Calm and clever Quarter Horses are great at working on cattle ranches.

Shetland (pony)

Shetland ponies are very strong. They have worked for people for hundreds of years.

Shetland ponies came from the Shetland Islands, off Scotland.

They even worked underground in mines, pulling heavy carts of coal through narrow tunnels.

Thick mane and tail

Thick winter coat

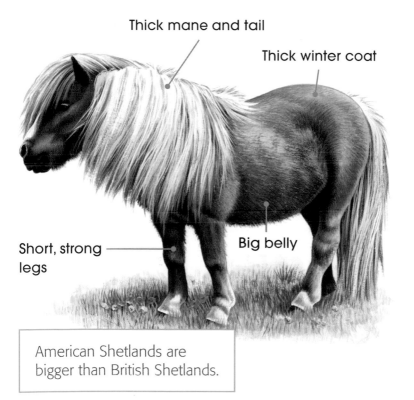

Short, strong legs

Big belly

American Shetlands are bigger than British Shetlands.

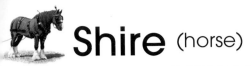

Shire (horse)

Before tractors and lorries were invented, farmers used horses to plough fields and pull heavy loads. Shires are the world's biggest, strongest horses.

Spot heavy horses showing off their skills at farm shows.

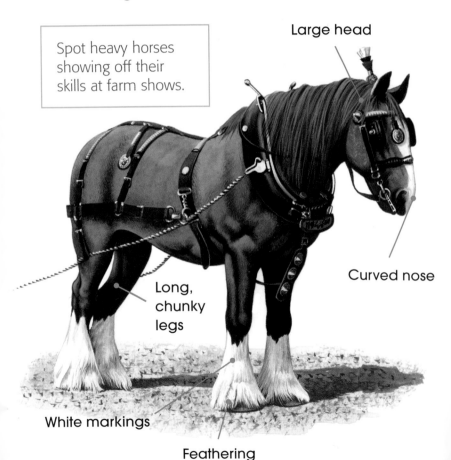

Large head

Curved nose

Long, chunky legs

White markings

Feathering

Skewbald and Piebald (horse)

Skewbald horses have patches of white and one other colour. Piebald horses have black and white patches. Their manes and tails also have two colours.

Skewbalds are usually white and brown.

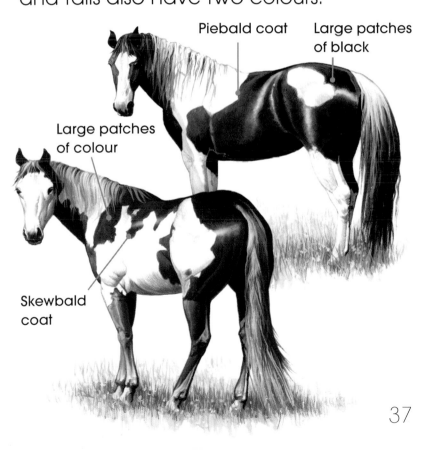

Piebald coat

Large patches of black

Large patches of colour

Skewbald coat

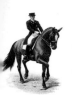

Swedish Warmblood (horse)

Swedish Warmbloods are popular riding horses. They are also brilliant at dressage, showjumping, and eventing.

Swedish Warmbloods have won medals at almost every Olympic Games.

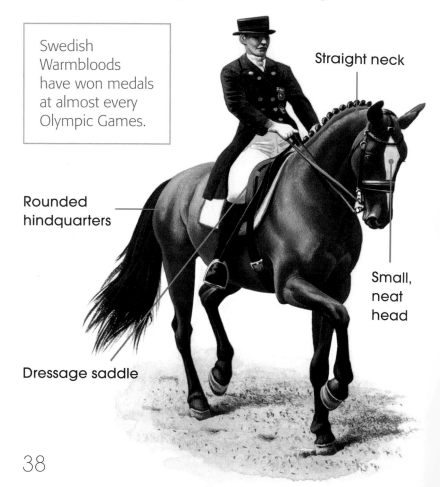

Straight neck

Rounded hindquarters

Small, neat head

Dressage saddle

Thoroughbred (horse)

These powerful horses are bred for racing. Thoroughbreds are popular in eventing and showjumping too. They can jump up to 10 metres – the length of two large cars.

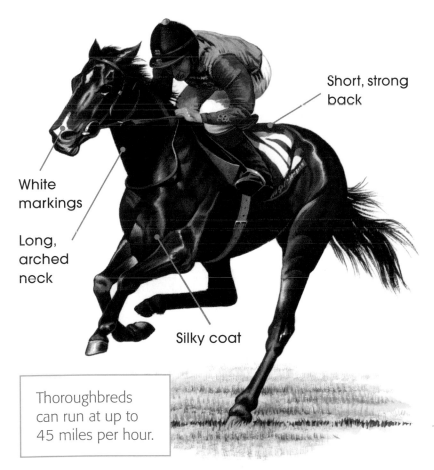

Short, strong back

White markings

Long, arched neck

Silky coat

Thoroughbreds can run at up to 45 miles per hour.

Welsh Pony and Cob (pony)

There are four types of Welsh Pony and Cob. Welsh Mountain Ponies are the smallest. You can see children riding them all over the world.

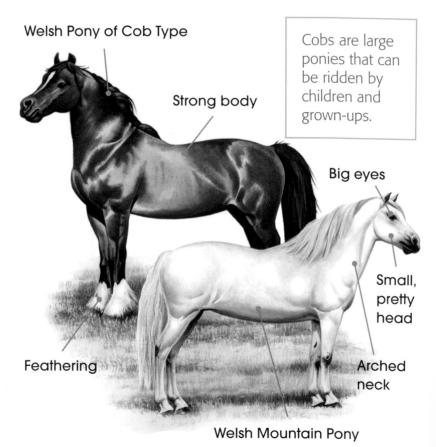

Welsh Pony of Cob Type

Strong body

Cobs are large ponies that can be ridden by children and grown-ups.

Big eyes

Small, pretty head

Arched neck

Feathering

Welsh Mountain Pony

Useful words

bay a brown horse with a black mane and tail. Some bay horses have a black muzzle, ears, mane, tail, and legs too

chestnut a reddish-brown horse with no black markings

dun a sandy-coloured horse with a black mane, tail, and lower legs. Most dun horses also have a dark stripe on their backs

equestrian sport a sport that tests the skills of a horse and rider, such as dressage and showjumping

gait the different ways in which a horse or pony moves

grey a horse with a coat that has mainly white hairs. Light-grey horses look white

hands the unit of measuring a horse or pony. One hand is the same as 10 cm (4 inches). The symbol hh means 'hands high'

heavy horse a large horse bred to pull heavy loads, or work on farms

hindquarters the back part of a
horse's body

light horse horses bred mainly for riding

palomino a horse with a golden coat
and a lighter mane and tail

pony all ponies measure less than
14.2 hands (142 cm). Camargues,
Caspians, Falabellas, and Przewalski's
Horses measure less than 14.2 hh, but
are usually called horses because of
their body shape and personality

roan a horse with a mixture of white
and coloured hairs in its coat

withers the highest part of a horse
or pony's back, between the
shoulder blades

Spotter's guide

How many of these horses and ponies have you seen? Tick them when you spot them.

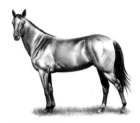

☐ Akhal-Teke
page 6

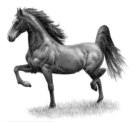

☐ American Saddlebred
page 7

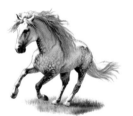

☐ Andalucian
page 8

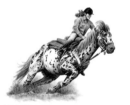

☐ Appaloosa
page 9

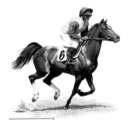

☐ Arabian
page 10

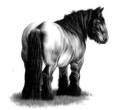

☐ Ardennes
page 11

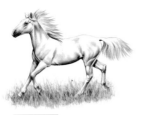

☐ Barb
page 12

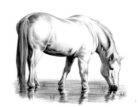

☐ Camargue
page 13

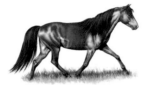

☐ Caspian
page 14

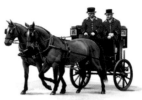

☐ Cleveland
Bay
page 15

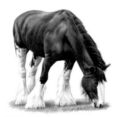

☐ Clydesdale
page 16

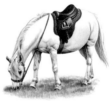

☐ Connemara
page 17

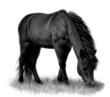

☐ Dartmoor
page 18

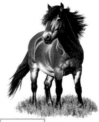

☐ Exmoor
page 19

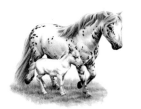

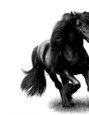

☐ **Falabella**
page 20

☐ **Fell**
page 21

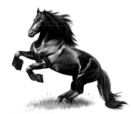

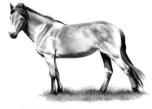

☐ **Friesian**
page 22

☐ **Gotland**
page 23

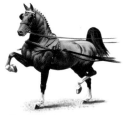

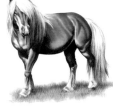

☐ **Hackney Horse**
page 24

☐ **Haflinger**
page 25

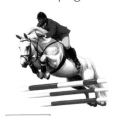

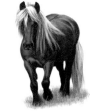

☐ **Hanoverian**
page 26

☐ **Highland**
page 27

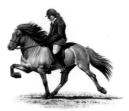
Icelandic
Horse
page 28

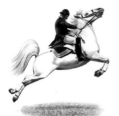
Lipizzaner
page 29

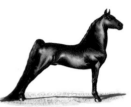
Morgan
page 30

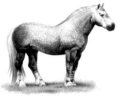
Percheron
page 31

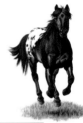
Pony of the
Americas
page 32

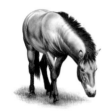
Przewalski's
Horse
page 33

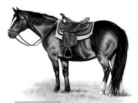
Quarter Horse
page 34

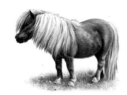
Shetland
page 35

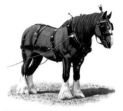

Shire
page 36

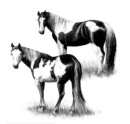

Skewbald and
Piebald
page 37

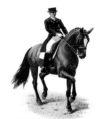

Swedish
Warmblood
page 38

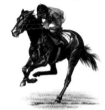

Thoroughbred
page 39

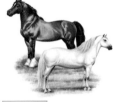

Welsh Pony
and Cob
page 40

Find out more

If you would like to find out more about horses and ponies, start with these websites. You will discover the different equestrian events, and find out where to watch horses and ponies in action.

The Pony Club
www.pcuk.org

The British Horse Society
www.bhs.org.uk

British Equestrian Federation
www.bef.co.uk

The British Show Pony Society
www.bsps.com

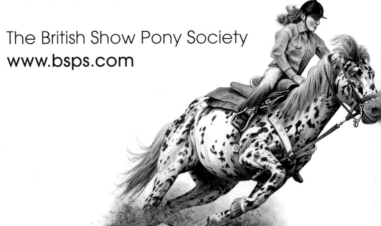